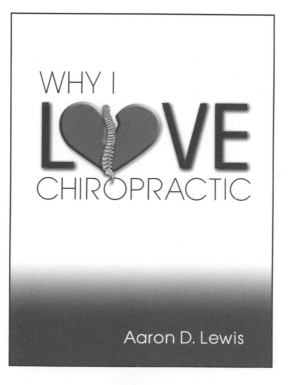

# WHY I
# L♥VE
## CHIROPRACTIC

Aaron D. Lewis

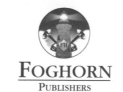

## FOGHORN
### PUBLISHERS
"Of Making Many Books There Is No End..."

Why I Love Chiropractic

ISBN-10: 1-934466-33-6
ISBN-13: 978-1-934466-33-9

Printed in China
©2010 by Aaron D. Lewis. All Rights Reserved.

Foghorn Publishers
P.O. Box 8286
Manchester, CT 06040-0286
860-216-5622
www.foghornpublisher.com
foghornpublisher@aol.com

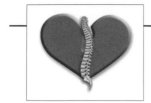

# Table of Contents

Introduction.......................................................... 1

1. Wrong Action, Wrongful Death...................... 7

2. The Miracle Within You ............................... 21

3. Don't Burn Down the House........................ 33

4. Dealing with Those Who
   Just Don't Understand.................................. 47

5. A Wellness Lifestyle ..................................... 59

About the Author ............................................. 73

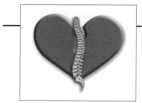

# Introduction

Right now I am sitting on Virgin Atlantic flight number 9 heading toward New York from London's Heathrow airport. At this point I'm ecstatic to be coming home—plumes of ash from the volcanic eruption in Iceland had grounded European air travel, and I was stranded in Belgium for two days on my way to the London Book Fair. Air travel wasn't the only affected transport; the Eurostar trains all over Europe had been booked solid since Friday and the show started Monday—but there wouldn't be a seat available until the following Wednesday. I suppose I could have taken a ferry, but those old boats were so overcrowded I'm still amazed they managed to stay afloat.

As bad as I thought things were for me, I realized when I looked around that so many people—full families of weary travelers—had it worse than I did. After all, I had somewhere to stay. I wasn't stuck in the airport for a week, sharing a back-breaking cot with a stranger, and eating whatever I could pull out of the vending machine. It was certainly an exercise in patience—I'll give it that. It was also educational, because I suddenly realized how much we—how much I—take for granted.

Each year I travel more than 100,000 miles to speak at events and offer consulting services, but until the flight restriction held me a veritable prisoner, I had given no thought to how truly amazing air travel actually is. I mean, I can go from New York to grabbing fish-and-chips in London in less than eight hours. I can get to Panama from New York in just five and a half hours, and that includes a one-hour layover in Miami. The point is that most people, like me, never realize how valuable and incredible something is until it's taken away for, say, a week or so.

Suddenly not having the freedom to fly made me appreciate air travel more than ever. Witnessing people sleeping among so many others at crowded departure gates reminded me that I could suffer worse than sleeping in a comfortable, private room. That some of those stranded travelers had curled up with thin blankets, their bodies trying to find comfort on a row of hard, plastic chairs, made me appreciate the luxury of a simple bed as I never had before.

And now, as I sit here in this airplane on my way home and watch people around me arching and bending, their movements accompanied by the sound of joints cracking, I know I must publicly express my appreciation for another underappreciated—and truly valuable—luxury: chiropractic.

I'm a firm believer that there is more than one way to do just about anything in life. All of the travelers stuck in Europe, and those waiting to get there, had several options. They could have taken a train or a ferry, they could have driven a car, or they might even have swum if they'd had the stamina of Michael Phelps.

The truth is, we all have options. Unfortunately, once we finally find the best option, we tend to forget just how amazing it is because we get so used to it that we take it for granted. Worse yet is when we haven't even discovered the better option, because we're stranded in a place of ignorance and ultimately left behind. In the case of chiropractic, not knowing about or utilizing it means we're not only left behind, but we're left behind in sometimes agonizing pain.

There were thousands of people stranded at the airport, sleeping in awkward positions on the floor or on chairs, the hours of discomfort no doubt wreaking havoc on their backs. I know they must have been in major pain, pain that could easily lead to other problems down the road. I thought, *Few of these people actually realize they don't have to adopt pain as a lifestyle.*

There are options. Have you given much thought to which option is best for you when it comes to back pain or pain in general? Is it drugs? Surgery? Although both conventional methods are the most widely accepted, personal experience, and the experiences of people I know, has convinced me that traditional methods aren't always necessarily the best methods.

When I discover a hidden jewel, I like to share it. This small book is not going to give you statistics, it's not a study in world medicine, and it won't provide fancy scientific research. This book is my way of sharing *Why I Love Chiropractic.* More than that, it's an opportunity for me to share why you should, too. I've figured out how to get rid of pain once and for all in a non-invasive way and live my life to the fullest, and it would be selfish of me to not try to help others with what I've learned.

With the healthcare system going through a complete upheaval as a result of America's determination to reform healthcare, and with the status of health declining globally, it is my duty to make you aware of what I think is one of the greatest treasures since the dawn of modern medicine. I believe that an open mind to a better way of healthcare may not only save you money, but it could possibly save your life. If it doesn't, I'm sure that it will at least change your perspective on life itself and the options we all have, but that we rarely consider.

# CHAPTER ONE

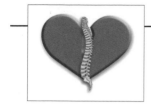

# Wrong Action, Wrongful Death

There are some people who fail to take action when they are sick and in pain, and others who take the wrong action because they don't know any better. Back in September of 1996, I was speaking at an event in Dallas, Texas, and on my second night there I received a phone call. My 37-year-old brother Derrick had died suddenly. It was late in the evening when I got the news, and afterward, I couldn't sleep. I was shocked not just by his death, but by how little sense it made. My oldest brother—"Ricky," as we affectionately called him—had always been the picture of perfect health.

He was the strong one, always lifting weights and flexing his muscles. His only weakness, if it could be called that, was that—like many—he had allergies. With or without them, he was my big brother, my hero. He was, I had thought, unbreakable. At dawn, I was using every bit of influence I had to get a seat on the earliest flight home. Fortunately, I was able to get a flight to Boston, which was only about 80 miles from my home in Connecticut. The trip was eerie,

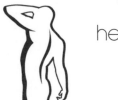

With or without allergies, he was my big brother, my hero. He was, I had thought, unbreakable.

because just a month prior to his death, Ricky had visited all of us with his family. I still vividly remembered riding on the back of his souped-up Yamaha 1100 motorcycle.

He'd just been right there, close enough for me to touch and alive and loving life; perfectly fit. I just couldn't make sense of why he had died so prematurely. When I got home, everyone was gathered together at my parents' house and making plans to fly out to Atlanta to finalize arrangements for my brother. When I got the chance, I took my hysterical mother aside to get the details surrounding Ricky's death. What I discovered was appalling. That summer, Ricky had been experiencing what he thought was an allergic reaction. His eyes were swollen and bloodshot red. His neck was engorged. He looked a mess, my mother said.

For as long as I could remember, Ricky had experienced allergies to such things as shellfish and tomato sauce, but he usually got over them as long as he avoided whatever triggered a reaction. It seemed logical that this latest flare-up was just another allergic reaction. Mother told me that Ricky, believing he had an allergy, went to the allergy specialist. A logical thing to do, right?

The doctor diagnosed my brother and gave him medication. Come to find out, my brother didn't have an allergy at all, but an overactive thyroid condition. The medication ended up acting like a deadly potion; it accelerated his thyroid's activity even more. So much so that it sped up his heart and caused him to have a heart

The greatest tragedy of it all is that his death could have been avoided.

attack. Imagine that. You go to the doctor to get better, and because of an incorrect diagnosis and steadfast adherence to traditional western medicine that discourages the exploration of other options, you die.

Ricky left behind a lovely wife and a young boy and girl. Yes, there was a wrongful-death lawsuit. After the lawyer got his commission of nearly half of the full award, Ricky's family was left with little to nothing, and Ricky was still gone.

The greatest tragedy of it all is that his death could have been avoided. It was after the lawsuit ended that I began my journey to wellness. I became a rebel with a cause, angry at the entire medical profession, and understandably so. The doctor who killed my brother with a quick and false diagnosis and fatal prescriptions is still practicing medicine, and I sometimes wonder how many other patients have been affected by the same blind faith in medicine and surgery that keeps them from searching for a better way.

## CHANGING YOUR ACTIONS CAN BRING LIFE

My first exposure to Chiropractic was nearly seven years ago. I was in Sarasota, Florida giving a motivational speech after spending weeks flying from place to place on business. Although I was fulfilled psychologically and emotionally after having had the opportunity to motivate and inspire so many, my body was not in the same good shape. I had piercing lower back pains that made it difficult to walk—my movements were slow and stiff. I've never liked to stretch much, so doing a series of stretches—even though it may have done something to alleviate a bit of the pain—was out of the question.

> He told me about things that were going on in my body that he couldn't possibly have known unless he were some kind of prophet.

Barring stretching, I had no idea there was actually a way for me to feel better. However, after my talk, I was approached by an ultra-aggressive chiropractor from Elmira, Ohio who told me how much he had enjoyed my talk. When, after talking for some time, I told him about my pain, Dr. Bob DeMaria told me that I was subluxated and that I needed an adjustment. I'd never heard that word in my life, and before I knew it, I was sitting in a big leather chair in the lobby of the Ritz Carlton being phys-ically evaluated by a dude I thought might be a little crazy.

He touched parts of my neck that were very sensitive. He'd ask, "Do you feel pain here?" Somehow, he knew I did. He was able to feel my pain, or at least locate it, with his fingers. And he could tell it hurt, because he'd touch a spot, and I'd suddenly shriek. Amazingly, with each area that was sore, he told me about things that were going on in my body that he couldn't possibly have known unless he were some kind of prophet. Or so I thought.

He could tell that I not only had tightness in my spine, but that I was also experiencing pain in my ears from frequent flights—and I hadn't even said anything to him about the pain in my ears. I was actually feeling pain in my ears right then and there. They hadn't popped in weeks, and everything sounded muffled. Dr. DeMaria asked me if I wanted an adjustment, and I didn't even know what an adjustment was. Because I had a medical mindset, I thought we would need to go behind closed curtains, or something, and that I would put on one of those open paper robes we've all worn at one time or another in doctors' offices.

I asked him if we needed to go to my room, but he told me that wasn't necessary and asked me to lie face down on the floor. He gave me a thorough adjustment right there, and it only took about ten minutes. The doctor then told me that I needed a lot of work. After I got up from the floor, he asked me to return to the leather chair, where he cracked my neck in both directions. The pop was so loud I thought he'd killed me—I guess I'd been watching too many Bruce Lee movies.

I wasn't dead, but from that moment on I did enter into a new life. I began walking a path that I would follow forever, because all of the pain in my lower back, the tension in my neck, and the pain in my ears disappeared—just like that. I wanted to take this curly-headed dude home with me, because I was certain he was the only one who had these magical powers. But then he told me about this secret treasure he called "chiropractic."

We talked for hours, well into the morning, about health and wellness and why so many people are not healthy. I started to get pretty angry, especially when he shared with me how so many people collectively rally against people in his profession because they are either ignorant, or they are afraid too many people will get

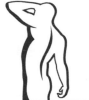

But then he told me about this secret treasure he called "chiropractic."

better and will no longer need the services of conventional doctors and conventional medicine. It was strange to me to realize there were so many millions of people who were sickened and diseased not because there was no help, but because they didn't know about chiropractic—or, worse, they didn't believe it would do them any good.

Even if they did believe it might work, too many simply didn't take any action, and simply believing won't get you very far in life if you don't take action. Some know about this treasure we call chiropractic, others are ignorant, and not enough are taking action. So, they stay ill.

I'M STARVING. PLEASE FEED ME.

The fact that people refuse to take action, reminds me of the story about the man who was dying from starvation. He hadn't eaten anything in several weeks and was close to death. He stumbled upon a hotel, and with the last bit of energy he could muster, he struggled through the doors, crying out for help, telling the first person he saw, "I NEED FOOD. I AM STARVING." With that, he finally collapsed. The attendant at the front desk panicked and called the medics. The starving man was getting worse by the minute as they waited for help to arrive.

Twenty minutes later, the paramedics were in the lobby examining the weak man. After about another ten minutes, the medic declared, "This man is dying of starvation. If he doesn't eat something fast, he will surely die." Immediately he asked the head chef to make the most nutritious meal he could within the next five minutes, as they were running out of time. Fortunately, it was dinnertime, and he was already close to completing the night's feast. In about five minutes, the head chef—dressed in white with the chef's hat to match—came running down the hallway from the kitchen and into the lobby.

With a smile and great enthusiasm, the chef announced his creation of six fabulous courses: chicken cordon blue with cous cous; sautéed garlic asparagus with brown sugar butternut squash; a large bottle of water; and crème brulée to top it off. The medic told the starving man, "If you eat some of this food, you will live." The tattered and fragile man said, "I DO BELIEVE I WILL LIVE IF I EAT THE FOOD." He kept saying it. "I DO BELIEVE I WILL LIVE IF I EAT THE FOOD."

He even got the medics and the hotel staff to start chiming in. "WE BELIEVE YOU WILL LIVE IF YOU EAT THE FOOD," they said. These mantras went on for about five minutes, and then everybody standing by witnessed the man taking his last breath before he died. A sad story, yet I only use this example to illustrate how so many of us could be so much better if we only ate the food we have before us. Sometimes the food is not actual food like steak or chicken or fresh vegetables and juice, but rather knowledge.

I hear the earth crying out for knowledge. However, what most people have been feeding on over the years is a bunch of garbage, garbage that keeps them in sickness and pain. If the man in the story had just eaten, he would have lived, but because he didn't eat, he died. Believing didn't do him a bit of good because he didn't follow through and act on his beliefs. Why do I love chiropractic? I love chiropractic because it teaches you *to live and not die.*

My brother wasn't like the starving man who refused to eat; he had taken action, but it was the wrong action, one that cost his life. Why do I love chiropractic? Because I believe that if my brother had been told to seek a second opinion and had been aware of the benefits of chiropractic, he might still be alive today. I believe chiropractic could possibly have saved my brother's life. I can hear it already—some of you reading this are saying, "There's no guarantee that your brother would have lived if he had seen a chiropractor. He could still have died."

You're right. He could have. But personal experiences and those of friends and loved ones I share in the pages to come will explain why I hold chiropractic in such high esteem. My brother chose the conventional path without giving something else a chance, and he lost everything. After losing him to such a poor choice, I swore I wouldn't go down the same path. I vowed to find a better way. Well, I found that way, and I'm sharing it with you.

# CHAPTER TWO

# The Miracle Within You

My greatest gifts are my five lovely children, all of whom receive regular chiropractic adjustments. My second daughter Amber is fifteen now, and she has suffered horribly with allergies ever since she was very young, most of the allergies associated with pollen during the spring months. Seeing my daughter suffer so badly was torture, and I felt it was my duty to help her find relief as quickly as possible. Because I didn't initially know any better, I simply thought all allergies were something people simply had to live with, and that there wasn't a natural way of dealing with allergic reactions.

All of the people who I knew who suffered from similar allergies would simply increase

...heir dosages of Benadryl or Claritin...get about 8-12 hours of relief. Every...would feel so bad for Amber as she strug...breathe through a stuffy nose and su...watery eyes and chronic itchiness. After...happened to my brother, I had little faith in d...tors, so I went to the natural health food store t...look for a natural pill, or herbal teas, or other...natural remedies. I did find both natural pills and herbal teas for her, but for whatever reason, she didn't get any better.

About this time, I'd been invited to speak on the topic of destiny at a few chiropractic events. I was scheduled to speak at an event at the Philadelphia airport, and I decided to take my daughter with me, just so she could hang out with her daddy. Initially, I thought I would speak and leave, as there were other speakers on the roster that weekend. I didn't really know how things were going to flow since I was new to the speaking circle. When I arrived, Doctors of Chiropractic had set up a "spinal fixit shop" in the middle of the ballroom floor with adjustment tables everywhere.

During the breaks, skilled doctors from all over America and Canada were practicing their techniques on one another. This was Amber's first time seeing anything quite like this, as she had never been exposed to chiropractic, and she was curious. Dr. John Madeira, the leader of the organization and the one who had invited me to speak, gave Amber an adjustment, and before we traveled back home, he had given her a couple more follow-up adjustments for the road. What would happen in the next few weeks impressed both my daughter and me, and it was nothing less than miraculous.

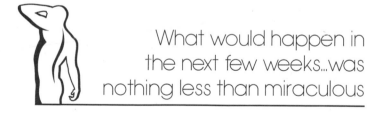

What would happen in the next few weeks...was nothing less than miraculous

Amber went through the rest of that spring and summer without any incidents of allergic reactions, despite the fact that that year saw the highest recorded levels of pollen during both spring and summer. This was the first time in four or five years that Amber was able to truly enjoy the spring without dreading the pollen and the furry white things that float around in the air, agitating her system. After that first allergy-free summer, Amber was hooked on chiropractic. Quite interestingly, if Amber doesn't get adjusted regularly these days, or if she's too busy to get adjusted, warning signs start to re-appear.

This goes to show how directly connected a well-adjusted spine is with total wellness—when her spine is properly adjusted, her major allergies

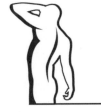

It really started to dawn on me that a healer is within each of us.

are altogether eliminated. There is obviously something going on inside of her body that requires adjusting in order to regulate her system in such a way that she can properly conquer her own allergies. It really started to dawn on me that a healer is within each of us. The healer is in you. The healer is in me. Chiropractic is simply the gift given to us to help strategically and safely activate the power within.

Amber never got to know her Uncle Ricky, but I often wonder what may have happened to Amber had I chosen the traditional route of going to an allergist. Perhaps she'd be with my brother. I'm not trying to sound overly critical of medicine, nor am I trying to horrify you with the facts concerning my brother's early departure from this world. I am knowledgeable enough to know that there has been much good done in the name of medicine over the years.

My contention is with the pervasive mindset of the majority, who automatically trusts every single bit of advice from medical doctors and finds no reason to question them. What people hear, they believe. No questions, no thinking. Before my brother's death, I was one of these people, too. But I've since learned how important it is to think, and to use our minds objectively. We don't have to believe everything we've been told about health, even if it is the conventional mindset. When it comes to life and death, we have to make educated choices. My brother never had the chance to learn the value of thinking outside of the box. But he gave that chance to me.

THE BODY CAN HEAL ITSELF

I've always been a firm believer that the body can heal itself. Yes, I believe an awesome creator was smart enough to equip us with a maintenance plan designed to keep our bodies working well. In the event that your system becomes depleted or broken down, you were designed with an internal repair kit called your nervous system. This system is a perfect system whose primary job is to keep you well. So, quite plainly, if your nervous system is out of order, your entire body will be out of order.

The nervous system is the most important part of your entire body; it controls all bodily functions. Now, like you, I believe in good hygiene. You should brush your teeth every day. Wash your face and clean behind those ears the way you were taught when you were young, and take a bath every day. My dentist always reminds me to floss after each meal to prevent tooth decay and gingivitis. All of those things are valuable parts of our daily routine. However, if I didn't bathe for a week, I'd still be alive and well.

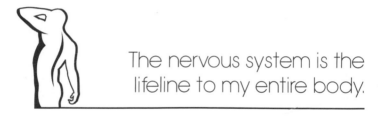

## The nervous system is the lifeline to my entire body.

If I didn't brush my teeth anymore, it is possible that I may get cavities and assault others with crazy bad breath, but I could still do the things I enjoy doing. I can live without teeth. I can live without a leg or even an arm, although I wouldn't want to do that. However, it is impossible for me to live without a spine. I cannot live without my nervous system. It is the lifeline to my entire body.

It is both a biblical principle and biological reality that there is life in the blood. You cannot live without blood, but worse yet, your blood has no idea what to do without a healthy nervous system giving it commands. Our entire body operates based on the commands and directives given to it by the nervous system.

## FREEING UP THE FLOW OF LIFE ENERGY

The spine is the lifeline to your entire body. Let me explain, according to my understanding, how regular adjustments made my daughter well. This is not a scientific explanation, but a recollection of the changes that occurred in my daughter as she went from an allergy sufferer pre-adjustment to someone who, post-adjustment, had no allergic reactions. Obviously, there was something in the environment that caused Amber to have an adverse allergic reaction. Maybe it was the pollen, or maybe it was something else carried by the wind.

In her system—and in yours, as well—there is something that, when her body is working properly, keeps Amber free from adverse reactions to pollen. It is an automatic defense mechanism that fights intrusive objects and substances that could irritate her system. But for some reason, whatever part of her nervous system that allows the free flowing movement of her natural internal allergy-fighters just wasn't receiving the right command. The fact that these internal fighters worked for her after an adjustment leads me to believe something was stopping the flow between her nervous system and whatever it is within her that fights the effects of pollen and other allergens.

In a sense, the chiropractor doesn't necessarily heal a person; the chiropractor simply frees up the clog in the system to make it work better so the body can heal itself. Look at the spine like it's a water hose. If I want to water my lawn so that it'll live and be beautifully green, my hose would need to be free of bends, and also clear of dirt and clogs, in order for the water to come out at full pressure. The longer the hose is clogged, the longer my lawn would have to wait to get watered.

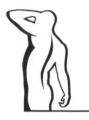

...the chiropractor frees the system so that the body can heal itself.

So, then, the probability of my lawn living and flourishing would be directly connected to how soon it could get watered. If I never fixed the clog, the lawn wouldn't receive water from the hose, and eventually my lawn would dry up and die. If I want my lawn to live, I have to unclog the hose. That is the same thing that happens in the human body. It dries up and dies when it does not receive the "watering," or the life energy, that comes through the hose we call the spine. The lawn, like our bodies, needs more than just water.

Water is of course a primary and essential nutrient, but it's only one of many things the lawn needs to be healthy. It also needs the right kind of soil. It needs sunshine. It needs oxygen, among other things. But if that one key element is not supplied—water—the lawn can die. Your nervous system supplies everything your body needs. So, then, it is extremely important to make sure your supplier is supplying. There may be something you are lacking or not being supplied, and in an extreme case, it may cause death—even as a result of a rushed misdiagnosis by a conventional doctor.

Less extreme cases may produce a lot of discomfort and pain. I'm convinced now more than ever that pain is a choice. The reason I say this is that you have a choice to do something about your pain to help correct it. And I'm not talking about surgery or medication. The chiropractor is the only doctor trained specifically to work with the spine to correct the problems in your body—or, as chiropractors would say, to correct the "subluxation" in your spine that may be causing tremendous pain or discomfort. When Amber's spine gets adjusted, her system is free to work optimally, allowing her body to do the work it was designed to do: heal itself.

This idea of allowing your body to heal itself using its innate and masterful design is not limited to just a few areas. Over the years, I have met several people who have suffered from pinched nerves, chronic back pain, headaches, endometriosis, scoliosis, neck pain, and weight problems, and who have all credited chiropractic care as the reason they have gotten well. Did chiropractic provide some kind of magical solution to the problem? No. It just opened the door that had been shut tight for many years, the door to their own personal healer within. You don't have to be drugged to death to get better. You simply have to give a chance to those who are trained to help you live your best life now.

# CHAPTER THREE

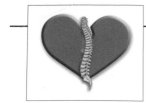

# Don't Burn Down the House

There are always alternative ways of doing things. Sometimes, however, those alternative ways go against the grain; they monkey with tradition. Let's face it, the most commonly accepted form of healthcare is taking medication, submitting to expensive scans and tests, or having a surgical procedure done if your medical doctor recommends it. I do not undervalue the role of a medical doctor; I realize that in cases of trauma or severe illness, a medical doctor is needed to provide emergency, or other specialized, care. However, medical doctors are not necessarily trained to keep me well.

Rather, they are trained to prescribe drugs and suggest treatments when they believe it is necessary, and I've come to discover that those "necessary" cases are not always necessary. When it comes to health, I believe it is of greater benefit to us to deal with the source of a prob-

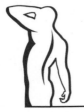

...medical doctors are not necessarily trained to keep me well.

lem than it is to approach the problem from an angle that focuses on the symptoms. What I appreciate about chiropractors is that they are far less likely to automatically attribute what may well be spine-related pain or numbness to the possible presence of an incurable disease, such as multiple sclerosis (MS) or amyotrophic lateral sclerosis (ALS, or Lou Gherig's Disease).

This is not to say the possibility of having such a disease doesn't exist, but a medical doctor will tend to lean too quickly in the "disease" direction, and chiropractors will first consider simpler reasons for the pain or numbness. Because they don't treat the symptoms doesn't mean they ignore them; chiropractors listen to the symptoms the client shares, and they then use that information as a way to try to find, and correct, the source of the problem. Also unlike conventional doctors, chiropractors don't treat. They don't ascribe to cures, and they surely don't medicate, because they believe the body knows how to heal itself given the right conditions.

The body will produce good health when treated correctly. What is a correctly treated body? A drug-free body. We have become a pill-popping society. There are pills for everything from stuffy noses to bad moods, and we take them to our detriment. Take, for example, what many of us do when we discover we have a fever: we take a pill to reduce it instead of allowing the body's higher temperature to do what it is suppose to do—fight the germs and chemicals causing the illness. I'm not saying an extremely high fever is healthy, or that there's no cause for concern.

What I am saying is that when the body heats up, taking a pill to reduce the fever in most cases only interferes with the process of natural healing. Prescription medication has its benefits. For instance, it treats infections. However, according to the article *Why Do Americans Take So Many Prescription Drugs?* by Dr. J. Douglas Bremner, Professor of Psychiatry and

> "Almost all of the chronic conditions for which pills are prescribed are preventable."

Radiology and Director of the Emory Clinical Neuroscience Research Unit (ECNRU) at Emory University School of Medicine in Atlanta, Georgia, "Almost all of the chronic conditions for which pills are prescribed are preventable."

Bremner concedes that "pharmaceuticals can be life saving for some conditions, such as insulin for Type I diabetes, thyroid hormone for hypothyroidism, or antibiotics for life threatening infections," but he also adds, "With so many of us popping pills or gulping down spoonfuls of medicine, it's not surprising that more of us report related adverse effects. One hundred thousand Americans die every year from the effects of prescription medications. Over a million Americans a year are admitted to the hospital because they have had a bad reaction to a medication. Many of these people are getting medications that they don't need, or for problems that can be appropriately and safely addressed without drugs."

Drugs do more treating of symptoms, and less healing of problems. In most circumstances, drugs simply suppress the sickness for a short while to provide temporary relief. Billions of dollars have been poured into medical research, yet we still have thousands of people dying each year of cancer, heart disease, lung failure, and other problems. It would seem like all of those dollars should, by now, have produced a cure, but it hasn't.

Being healthy means being more concerned with creating a lifestyle of wellness than with succumbing to a lifestyle of drug-induced escapism. Chiropractic is another way, a better way. We just have to overcome the temptation to stick with what we've been programmed by hundreds of commercials and magazine ads to believe—that we need more drugs and more medical procedures, and very little exploring of the healing methods found outside of the box.

## NO SURGERY FOR ME

In addition to mentoring my five children, I am also a mentor and father figure to others, one of whom is a very special young lady, Jasmine Brown, to whom I have been a mentor since she was six years old. She is now 18, and she's in good health, but when Jasmine was 13, she went to her school nurse for a routine check-up at her middle school. The nurse noticed that she had a pretty noticeable curve in her spine, and she sent Jasmine home with a note to her mother suggesting that she see a doctor to confirm her findings.

Jasmine and her mother, JoAnna, visited her primary care doctor, and she too confirmed that Jasmine had a significant curve in her spine, and she said it needed immediate attention. Her recommendation was that Jasmine have surgery to correct the problem right away, as it would quickly worsen. She referred her to an orthopedic specialist who could verify the need for surgery and offer further advice. This seemed a bit strange to both Jasmine and her mother. Jasmine is a bubbly soul and an energetic athlete. She never complained of any back pain or discomfort.

Jasmine was starting guard for both her school basketball team and the AAU (Amateur Athletic Union) traveling basketball team, and she had high hopes of someday playing college ball and perhaps playing professionally for the WNBA after college. The orthopedic specialist took several x-rays and found that Jasmine had a 38-degree curve in her spine spreading from her lower to middle lumbar. They told her quite honestly that her condition would definitely worsen over time and there wasn't anything they could do to completely correct the problem. They did say, however, that although surgery wouldn't correct the problem, it would prevent it from advancing.

The doctors told Jasmine that if the curve continued to increase, it would eventually curve until her body contorted to such a degree that she would be bent over sideways. If that happened, Jasmine would be deformed for the rest of her life, her hopes of playing collegiate basketball or having the kind of future she envisioned destroyed. The doctor gave her two options: surgically insert pins into her spine to help prevent it from curving further, or wear a custom-made brace to try to retain the curve and at least slow the inevitable process.

I remember the two of them talking to me about this problem, as well as my suggestion that they consider alternate options. But definitely, I said, do not allow them to cut "Miss Jasmine," as I love to call her. JoAnna and Jasmine chose the back brace, believing it to be the lesser of the two evils. Jasmine began wearing the brace 23 hours of each 24-hour day, and from the very onset she hated it with a passion. The doctors recommended she wear it for three years, but depending on how well she acclimated to the brace, it could go on for much longer than that.

The doctors reasoned that since she was only 13 and was still growing steadily, her curve would grow with her. I remember seeing Jasmine after she'd begun wearing the brace, and it was the first time I'd seen her—this spirited girl who had always seemed to have a reason to smile— looking so unhappy. She complained that the brace was stiff and hard, and that it bent her body to the side. She felt overly conscious of having to walk awkwardly as not to appear to be walking sideways.

She hated wearing it even more during the summer months. She could only wear certain shirts with it, and she also had to wear extra clothing if she wanted to try to disguise it (which she did). The brace, the t-shirt she wore over it, and the t-shirt she wore over the t-shirt to hide the brace, kept her hot and sweaty through the summer. Many times, she simply took off the brace against the doctor's wishes just to get a day or two of relief. What Jasmine didn't know is that her mother was already looking for alternatives and had been researching chiropractors.

Her doctor was extremely resistant to the idea of giving a chiropractic recommendation. When JoAnna asked the doctor if chiropractic would help, she never explicitly said anything for or against chiropractors, but she was very slow to give a recommendation. Finally, after much insistence, JoAnna managed to get a referral. The two saw the chiropractic doctor, who said he had seen many cases like Jasmine's. He suggested that she begin to get regular adjustments—at least three times weekly—and JoAnna told her daughter she had to continue to wear the brace while getting those regular adjustments.

The chiropractor said he couldn't promise the adjustments would fix Jasmine 100%, but he did promise her situation would improve, and that she wouldn't need surgery. Jasmine, realizing that she had found a better way and in a hurry to be rid of the brace, began to cheat a bit more...she only wore the brace intermittently. The amazing thing was that, even after not following instructions and taking off the brace more often than she should have, her spine still went from a 38-degree curve to a 31-degree curve within months of beginning her adjustments. Today, five years later, her spine is even better.

Surgery—one of the first options presented by medical doctors—was not an option for her, nor did it need to be. Luckily, Jasmine's mother thought to ask about the possibilities of chiropractic care. Before giving it a try, JoAnna didn't know very much about it, but she did know that it was a possible way to help her daughter avoid surgery, and that was enough for her. She thought, "Id rather try that than try nothing."

Today, Jasmine is an exceptional student at Mt. Holyoke College, and yes—her dream of playing college basketball has become a reality. She is still getting regular adjustments, and her life is looking good.

# A LITTLE MOUSE AND A BURNED DOWN HOUSE

Suppose you had a mouse problem in your house that persisted for quite some time, and you finally reached the breaking point; it was time to do something about it. How many options would you have? Let's see...you could hire a professional pest control specialist. It would be a bit pricier than if you tried to manage the invasion yourself, but it's an option. The specialists would come in and set up traps for the mouse, and maybe after a week or so they would come back, collect the dead mouse, and send you the bill.

As mentioned above, you could do it yourself. The frugal crew—and I know this, because I'm frugal, too—loves this option, because it's cheap and often effective. You just go down to your local hardware store, purchase a mousetrap, and follow the instructions. In perhaps the same amount of time as it takes the professionals, you'll trap the mouse. (Of course, if you are afraid of mice, this may not be the best choice, because you'll have to be the one to do all of the clean-up work.)

Another option is to get a cat. Cats eat mice, if you can find a cat that likes to hunt. And not all cats do. Even if they do, the mouse will often run away from the cat or will simply vacate the premises—leaving the territory open for a new mouse to occupy. Just the presence of a cat will usually solve your problem with the least bit of trauma to you, your household, and your budget, but you also have to want to (and be able to) take care of a cat.

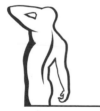

When you get surgery you are destroying your "house."

Or, hey—you could just douse your house with gasoline and light it with a torch. Burn the whole thing down. Of course, there's no guarantee you'll get rid of the mouse, but you sure will have done a number on your house. Unfortunately, millions of people choose to destroy their own house—their body. They do this when they make uninformed decisions based on poor suggestions from closed-minded, or profit-minded, professionals or the barrage of advertisements and drug endorsements they see on television, all of them recommending that they take medication, or have procedures performed that could destroy the entire body.

Drugs can destroy your "house." When you get surgery, you are destroying your "house." You may be alleviating the effects of the problem, but at the same time, you're getting rid of yourself in the process. Had Jasmine and Joanna followed the doctor's recommendation to have a surgical procedure done, Jasmine would not only have severely damaged her "house," but she would also have shattered her dreams in the process.

Your life, your dreams, and your body are far too important to entrust it all to a single health philosophy, as popular as that philosophy may be. Remember, there are many ways to conquer a problem. Chiropractors are trained to help you address your problem without burning down your house.

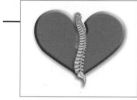

# CHAPTER FOUR

# Dealing with Those Who Just Don't Understand

I have always believed in compassion, and I do my best to present myself in a way that shows compassion, especially to those who are unaware of some of the things I often mistakenly think are common knowledge. But showing compassion isn't always easy to do. Anything that has the potential to produce good in this world will always be attacked. That's just one of life's realities. And it can often be quite difficult trying to reason with people who are unreasonable, or who have an ulterior motive, or who may just be brainwashed by a system inadvertently designed to kill us.

Jesus was killed for healing the sick and offering salvation; Ghandi, who only wanted to pursue peace, was assassinated on his way to address a prayer meeting; Nelson Mandela was imprisoned for decades for opposing the South African system of apartheid; Rev. Dr. Martin Luther King Jr. was jailed, beaten, and imprisoned for rallying for civil rights and racial equality. So it isn't so strange that chiropractors are attacked in the media, and especially by the medical profession, if they are offering a better way.

> Their interest isn't promoting health, but promoting illness, because illness is BIG BUSINESS.

Most people realize that the pharmaceutical companies earn billions of dollars through drug sales. Medical doctors earn tremendous amounts of money, incentives, and commission overrides every time you use a drug they've recommended. Plenty of doctors work hand in hand with pharmaceutical companies to ensure they both make a profit. Their interest isn't promoting health, but promoting illness, because illness is BIG BUSINESS. Knowing this makes it easier to understand why some medical doctors and the drug industry at large would want to publicly question the credibility of chiropractors. It's just common sense. If more people get well, the drug companies will have a major drop in profit.

The more people who are well, the greater the drop in need for surgeries. It's all about the money. You and I are simply the pawns. We are being preyed on, and the predators' first objective is to make us believe our friend—the chiropractor, in this case—is actually our enemy. They make horrible and unsubstantiated claims about chiropractors because, I believe, they sense their own days are numbered. Quite simply, healthcare as we knew it is dying a steady death. When it does finally collapse, people like you and me will have to consider other avenues, and the roads less traveled will become a less surprising direction for us.

Before that time, though, you still have to run for your life and protect your number one investment—YOU. If you want to become a fool in life, try reasoning with a fool. You, too, will become one. There are some people I know will not see reason, and so I refuse to spend my time trying to force it on them. They won't listen no matter how valid my argument is, so I don't bother. But then you have those people who aren't fools, but who are just influenced by the onslaught of very effective propaganda and clever media using fear to encourage people in one direction or another.

Yes, FEAR is the greatest motivator. How unfortunate it is that people will use fear, perhaps the most debilitating of emotions, to get you to do things you did not plan to do. A few years ago, on Super Bowl weekend, the weather forecasters predicted one of the worst storms ever to hit Connecticut. They forecasted at least four feet of snow. They told the people, "You better be prepared. This is going to be the big one." Choosing responsibility over luxury, thousands of unenthusiastic men returned their big screen televisions—high def, even—so they would have money to buy snow blowers.

Well, the Super Bowl came and went. Football fans struggled to watch the game on tight screens. And it never snowed. Not a flake. Quite naturally, everyone with new snow blowers and tiny televisions were pretty ticked off, because they bought into the fear the media told them they should have. I'm here to ask you not just to be open to a better way, but to also be open to the possibility of big businesses trying to use fear to steer you where they want you to go. Maybe if you're given some of the popular arguments in advance, you'll be better prepared for the foolishness and mudslinging if it comes your way.

## COMMON ARGUMENTS AND HOW I'D DEAL WITH THEM

Opponents of chiropractic might say something like, "They manipulate your spine." First, chiropractic is not about the manipulation of the spine, but rather the gentle adjusting of the spine. I've been adjusted a number of times, and my chiropractor, Dr. William Bazin, has never manipulated my spine. He's never hurt me or caused me pain. If he did manipulate my spine, I'm sure it would be in such bad shape that it would warrant this technique. For the most part, however, spine manipulation is not a common practice for the chiropractor. And if it were, I have to say—I'd much rather chiropractors manipulate my spine than have drug industries manipulate my mind.

> I'd much rather chiropractors manipulate my spine than have drug industries manipulate my mind.

Another opinion is that chiropractic is not scientific. Here again we have given far too much leeway to medical science to determine what is science from what it is not. Science is simply, according to standard definition, "a systematic study of the structure and behavior of the physical and natural world through experiment." Not only does chiropractic fall under this definition, but it can also be called an art because chiropractors perform their care through the artistic and skilled guidance of their gifted hands, knowledgeably placing them where they need to go to produce results.

My question is: does one have to understand science in order to enjoy its benefits? You enjoy the benefits of electricity, air travel, and even breathing fresh air every day, but if I were to ask you to write a ten page paper explaining how all of those things work, unless you were trained in those disciplines, you probably wouldn't be able to explain it to me until you did some research. Nonetheless, with or without your understanding, those scientific benefits are what they are. The general lack of understanding when it comes to chiropractic philosophy doesn't mean it is any less scientifically based, or any less effective.

Some might say to worry if a chiropractor seems too confident or overzealous about chiropractic care. Okay. I know this is a book, but I have to take a moment, here, because that has to be the most irrational argument I've ever heard. Why would anyone not be enthusiastic about what they do? If my chiropractor had no zeal about his own profession, I wouldn't want to be bothered with it as a patient. Overzealousness is not a reason to scrutinize your chiropractor.

> The job of the chiropractor is to offer a natural alternative to medicine.

What you should beware of, however, is a chiropractor who does not disparage regular medication. The job of the chiropractor is to offer a natural alternative to medicine, so they have no logical reason not to expose the drugs that may be the cause of sicknesses growing in you. Alternatively, this explains why the conventional medical community doesn't offer chiropractic as an alternative. Would the drug dealer promote regular exercise as the way to get a high in life? The owner of a chain of gyms wouldn't say, "Hey, if coming to my gym doesn't work, you can always use cocaine to get high."

Wellness doctors are *supposed* to criticize prescription drugs, especially those that have been proven to cause harm to the body. There are so many ridiculous claims against chiropractors—far too many to list—and doing it will only waste paper and space, anyway. Writer and newspaper editor Leo Aikman once said, "You can tell more about a person by what he says about others than you can by what others say about him." What's important is not what others say about chiropractic, but what chiropractic can do for you. Also important is to become more interested in questioning motives.

Chiropractic has never been proven to harm anyone. In fact, medical associations and private medical practices directly funded the few chiropractic scares that have been promoted on the news and placed on billboards. That is what I call a questionable motive. The impetus behind such a strategic assault was not the promotion of health and wellbeing, but the preservation of their professions, which are becoming increasingly expensive due to enormous malpractice insurance costs and wrongful death lawsuits, such as the one filed after the death of my brother.

The drug companies bombard me every day of my life with some subtle or overt form of attempted mind control, but not once have I felt manipulated by a chiropractor. Your spine is fine in the hands of the chiropractors; that's what they were trained to do. Some people don't understand their value. Others understand, yet they reject the information because they are either afraid to try something new, or they've been convinced by the media, or they're part of the big business medical and pharmaceutical giant and, consequently, have a hidden agenda.

Don't let the detractors of chiropractic care convince you so easily that the practice isn't legitimate. Instead, if you have questions, call a chiropractic office. Talk to some people who have visited a chiropractor. Do what we should all do when making any important medical decision: research. The best way to deal with ignorance is through education. But again, you can only educate those who will accept the knowledge. This book is one way to begin the process of learning a better way. There are many educational and informative resources available online and in print that will provide even more understanding about wellness living.

No one paid me to write any of this. In fact, there isn't a chiropractor in the world who knows I'm writing this book right now. I intentionally kept my plans quiet until it went to the presses, and I didn't ask for any endorsements from any chiropractors. I simply wanted you, and everyone else who would read this book, to be aware that there is great gift available to you, but if you don't know to look for it, it will pass you by. Don't take my word for it, though. Research it for yourself.

You may decide you don't have an interest in seeing a chiropractor, and you may decide you can live and enjoy a more pain-free life by making a few simple adjustments. (No pun intended.) Either way, the decision is yours—but until you are aware of all of your options, there is little to decide.

*My people are destroyed from lack of knowledge. "Because you have rejected knowledge, I also reject you." —Hosea*

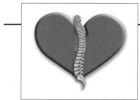

CHAPTER FIVE

# A
# Wellness Lifestyle

The foundation of chiropractic can be summed up in one word—wellness. Wellness, however, is not something one strives for every now and again, but is a way of life. What is wellness? Wellness is a healthy state of wellbeing free from sickness and disease. Wellness is also wholeness in your family life, your spiritual life, your emotional state and your physical aptitude. You can be free from sickness and disease, yet carry grudges toward people you refuse to forgive. In time, that negative energy, those harsh emotions will catch up with you and may allow sickness to creep into your body.

In 2003, CBS reported on a study performed by Ohio State University researchers Janice

Kiecolt-Glaser and her husband Ronald Glaser that suggests "a chemical called Interleukin-6 sharply increased in the blood of the stressed.... Previous studies have associated IL-6 with several diseases, including heart disease, arthritis, osteoporosis, type-2 diabetes and certain cancers." Wellness truly is a state of mind; it is a condition of your heart and soul. Even though chiropractors deal with the nervous system and

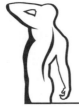

Wellness truly is a state of mind; it is a condition of your heart and soul.

regular adjustments are its primary delivery of wellness, they do not ignore the fact that there are many other areas that can also influence your health.

Their objective is to help you to cover all of the bases, and my purpose is to try to get you to understand how living a healthy lifestyle—

being an active participant in your life—is more than being a reactive participant who tends to the body only when it's not well. Most people are prone to care about their health a lot more when they have a traumatic emergency or when they just feel like crap, but I'm here to try to convince you to do what you can to avoid getting to that point.

It is far easier to learn how to think like a healthy person and take the necessary steps toward living a healthy lifestyle. In order to do this, you will have to erase the program living in your consciousness that has you accepting sickness as a lifestyle. Our media, and our society, programs us in a number of ways— not the least of which is with its prescription drug advertisements—to expect sickness and welcome it into our lives as if it's a normal thing. There are billboards all around my city promoting the best local cancer doctors and heart specialists.

Now, I understand that people who suffer from various issues need to know who they can go to for help, but I can't get past how powerfully their messages seem to be promoting sickness rather than health. What message do we internalize when the ads and the billboards say, "What if you get sick?" instead of "Walk in health"? When you see yourself as well, and when you view wellness as a likely option for your life, you will begin to make choices that will support a healthy lifestyle all the time, rather than whenever you're reminded by an illness—or the fear of it.

## GET ADJUSTED REGULARLY

The first thing I will emphasize is that you need to get adjusted regularly. I've spoken with people over the years who tried chiropractic, and who have then said to me, "I don't know, Lewis. I went to the chiropractor once or twice, and my condition isn't getting any better. That junk don't work." I'd immediately ask them, "Are you hungry?" They'd of course say, "Yeah, I'm a little hungry. So? What's that got to do with anything?" I'd say, "Well, you shouldn't be hungry because you've eaten once or twice this week, haven't you?" And they would say, "Man, that's different."

Actually, it isn't any different at all. Your body needs to "eat" regular adjustments to keep things functioning right. Perhaps not as much as

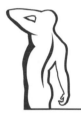

Get on a maintenance plan and be seen on a regular basis.

we all eat—three adjustments a day would be excessive—but it does need nutrients on a regular basis in order to be strong and healthy. You wouldn't eat one meal this year and think it'd suffice. You wouldn't take one bath and hope that it keeps you fresh for the entire month. You wouldn't take one college class and think you've mastered a subject. Why, then, should you believe that after one adjustment your health should show any major improvements?

It's true that some people have had an adjustment or two and have felt remarkably better afterward. That's not abnormal. But in order to continue feeling that way, you're going to have to get on a maintenance plan and be seen on a regular basis. Consistency breeds success, and not just in people. My piano goes out of tune—I have to get it tuned three or four times annually. If I'd only tuned it two or three times in the decade I've owned it, not only would it sound horrible, but it would also be damaged from lack of proper care. People aren't any different from my piano—think of a chiropractor as the tuner of your spine. Getting adjusted is the first step toward wellness, as a healthy spine supports all of your other health efforts.

EATING PROPERLY

This is always a touchy area, because people love to eat whatever they want to eat. And in fact, eating is a very cultural thing, so I don't want to touch this old taboo topic. What I will say, though, is that whatever you are eating right now, just use your commonsense-wellness mindset to start making more healthy choices. Believe it or not, many people don't know what they should eat from what they shouldn't. And if you are one of those people, I recommend doing a little research about the proper balance of food groups for your body type.

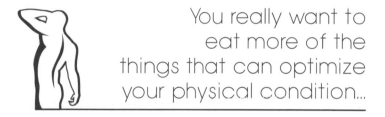

You really want to eat more of the things that can optimize your physical condition...

As a rule of thumb, you should eat more fruits and green leafy vegetables, as they are an important source of nutrients and help to aid in healthy digestion. Whole foods, as they are called, can help lower cholesterol and high blood pressure. You really want to eat more of the things that can optimize your physical condition and, as a general rule, stay away from a whole lot of fried foods, sodas, and sugar-filled foods.

Finally, drink more water. It doesn't matter how much I tell you to drink a day, because you're probably not going to drink that much, anyway. Just drink more than you do now, okay? These small steps, once implemented, will eventually become routine and will help you develop a wellness mindset. It won't happen overnight, but neither does bad health. It happens over time, and you can use time as your friend or foe.

## EXERCISE

Develop an exercise plan you will actually stick with. It really doesn't matter what it is, as exercise is very much based on personal preference. I particularly enjoy cycling outdoors, running, rowing, and working out on the elliptical trainer. I run marathons, but I obviously don't expect everyone reading this book to join me. Some people just hate running. You may like walking, stretching, playing tennis, or even swimming. Nowadays, you can even get decent exercise playing the Wii, with games especially designed to increase physical activity. Whatever you like to do, just do it, and keep doing it until long after you get the results you desire so you can maintain those results. Getting exercise keeps your bones, heart, and muscles strong.

## ENVIRONMENT

One thing so many fail to consider as something requiring our care is our own planet. The way you treat the earth will have an incredible impact on your personal life and your own well-being. The saying goes, "There is no debt in the universe that will go unpaid." When you destroy the earth, you destroy yourself. There is a direct parallel between the condition of the earth and the condition of her inhabitants.

Get more involved with initiatives to promote clean water and clean air throughout your community, and if you have the means, go abroad. Get to know your planet—it's a lot bigger than the country you're familiar with. You don't have to travel to become acquainted, though;

when you were a child, you played under trees, dug into soil, climbed rocks, and walked alongside rivers or streams. Get to know the earth again—plant a tree, a bush, or even a small shrubbery. If you haven't already, start recycling.

Do things to demonstrate that you care about your world and the condition it's in. I've come to realize that the people who are most

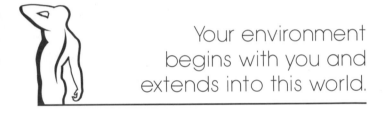

Your environment begins with you and extends into this world.

concerned about the world in which they live are also concerned about the body in which they live. Your environment begins with you and extends into this world. Everything moves from the inside out, not the other way around. However you treat your body (supposing that you treat it well), begin to treat your environment the same way. This is the process of cultivating a wellness mentality.

## HAVING A TIME FOR PRAYER AND MEDITATION

Wellness thinking has much to do with the physical body, but it also has a lot to do with your spirit. You can have a healthy physical body, but also have a decaying spirit. Anything you do not use will eventually die from lack of use. For example, if I chose not to use my arm and refused to move it for the next ten years or so, the muscle would turn to goop. My arm would atrophy. I have to move my arm every day in order for it to be fully functional, fully alive.

In the same way, you need to take time out for prayer or simply give thanks or recognition to all of the things you have in your life. Take time out to express your gratitude for all of your many blessings. If you feel like you don't have much to be thankful for, you can start by just expressing gratitude for the fact that you are alive. Be thankful for life—not everyone has had it for as long as you have, you know.

Learn how to meditate, an exercise I believe is an extension of prayer.

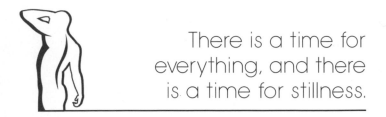

There is a time for everything, and there is a time for stillness.

Learn to quietly think and contemplate and be grateful for where you have come from, and also where you are going. It's in these quiet times that you begin to discover your greater self and cultivate a greater awareness about yourself, others, and the universe around you. Life can be stressful. And bad stress will lead to bad health. A wellness mindset comes more easily when time is taken to just be quiet—to just be. There is a time for everything, and there is a time for stillness.

Take the time now. Appreciate all that you have, all that you are, and all that your magnificent human body has been designed to do. Your mind, your organs, your muscles, and your spine all work together when they're healthy as a brilliant and miraculous system, and this alone is a blessing to be grateful for. I believe that as you develop a wellness mentality you will discover a new place of healthfulness, wholeness, and peace in your life, something that has always been closer to you than you knew before, and with this, you will be less inclined to put all of your faith in drugs and conventional medicine, because you will better know the power of your own body, as well as its limitations, and you will have the confidence to be the judge of what treatment is best for you.

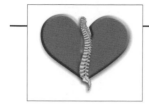

# About the Author

Aaron D. Lewis is a spiritual leader, humanitarian, the ghostwriter of more than 100 books, and a consultant to major publishers in the United States and Europe. He lives in New England and Panama.

To learn more about the author, visit:
www.whyilovechiropractic.com
www.thescribesink.com
www.4ghostwritersonly.com

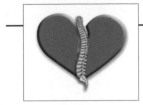

# Also by Aaron D. Lewis

BOOKS

Healing for the 21st Century

Keys to Unlocking Your Destiny

The Total Package: Keys to Acquiring Wealth and Walking in Divine Health

The Obama Principle: Creating a Life of Reward Through the Power of Perseverance

SHORT STORY

Searching for Solutions

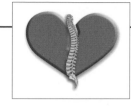

# To Order
# Why I Love
# Chiropractic

To order your own copy of *Why I Love Chiropractic,* or if you are a chiropractor interested in placing a bulk order, please call 860-216-5622.

Or visit us online at www.whyilovechiropractic.com

## FOGHORN
### PUBLISHERS
"Of Making Many Books There Is No End..."